THIS BOOK

BELONGS TO

....

....

Is Spinach Dip Healthy? Here's What a Dietitian Says

Spinach dip is a tasty, easy-to-make dip that's a perfect party food or appetizer for a crowd.

Still, not all spinach dips are created equal. Some are calorie-dense and contain a lot of saturated fat and sodium while others are lighter, filled with vegetables, and offer healthy fat and protein.

Both store-bought and homemade spinach dips can be healthy or unhealthy depending on the ingredients and what foods you serve it with.

This article explores spinach dip's nutrients, benefits, and drawbacks, as well as tips for making your own healthy version.

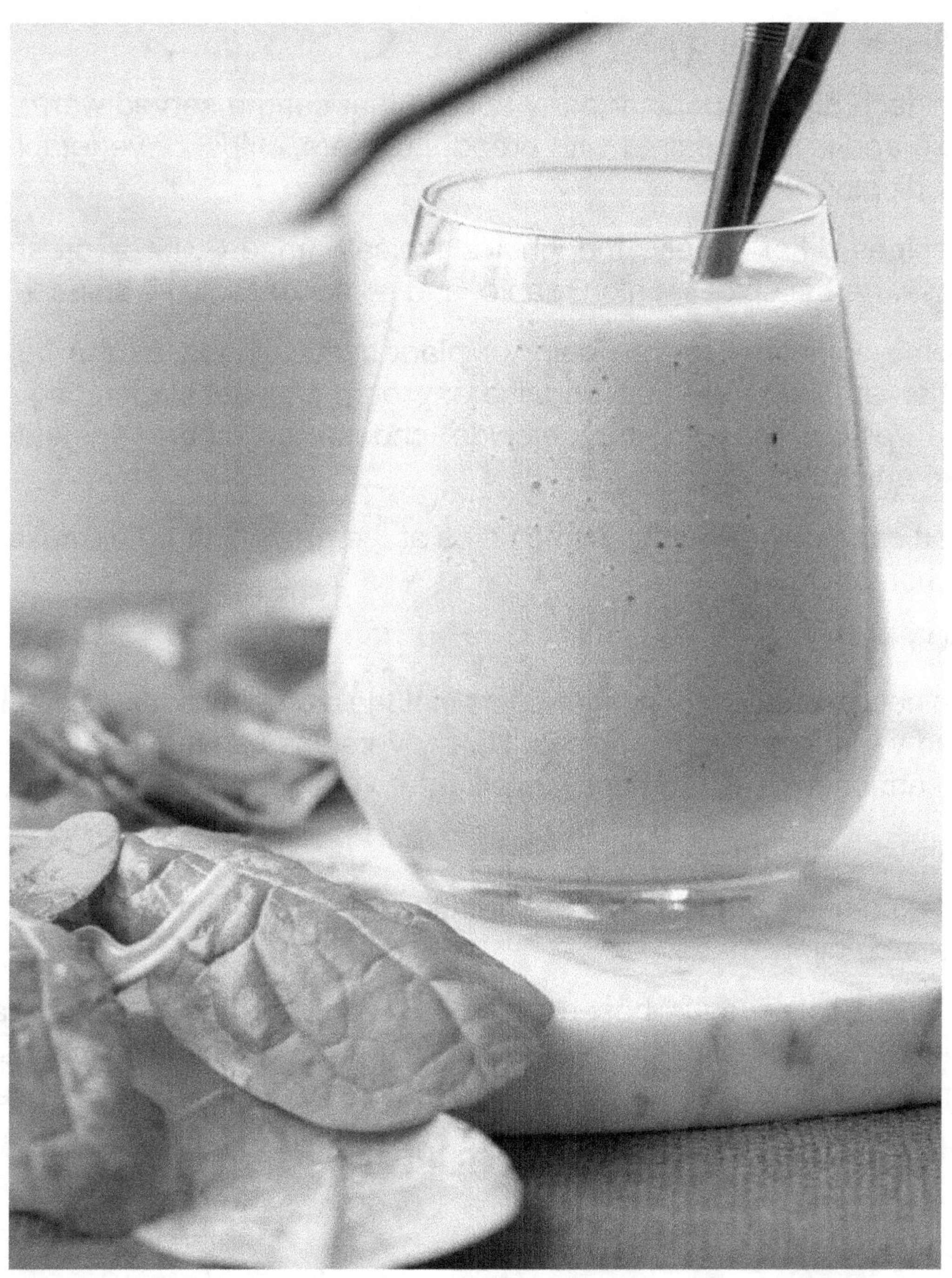

What is spinach dip?

Spinach dip is a popular party spread that can be served warm or cold and is often paired with bread, crackers, chips, or vegetables for dipping.

Recipes differ widely, though it's typically made with a creamy base, herbs, spices, onion, garlic, and — necessarily — spinach.

Some spinach dips use dairy or plant-based yogurt as the base whereas others use mayonnaise or cream cheese. Depending on the recipe, the dip may include cheese or other vegetables like artichokes.

You can buy pre-made spinach dips at the grocery store or make it at home.

SUMMARY

Spinach dip's common ingredients include a creamy base, spinach, and various herbs and spices. Heavy versions use mayonnaise or cream cheese as the base while lighter versions may use yogurt.

Spinach dip nutrition

The calorie count and other nutrition facts depend on how the spinach dip is made.

For example, yogurt-based dips boast more protein and less fat than a mayonnaise or cream-cheese based dip. Adding cheese and oils will add fat, including some saturated fat from the cheese.

Nutrition facts for basic spinach dip recipes

The following chart outlines the nutrition facts for 2 tablespoons (30 grams) of homemade spinach dip made with yogurt, regular mayo with sour cream, or light mayo with light sour cream

	Yogurt and mayonnaise spinach dip	Regular mayo and sour cream spinach dip	Light mayo and sour cream spinach dip
Ingredients	frozen spinach, low fat plain Greek yogurt, mayonnaise, salt, milk	frozen spinach, milk, mayonnaise, sour cream, salt	frozen spinach, light mayonnaise, light sour cream, milk, sugar, salt
Calories	48	100	50
Protein	2 grams	less than 1 gram	less than 1 gram
Total fat	4 grams	11 grams	4 grams
Saturated fat	1 gram	2.5 grams	1 grams
Carbs	1 gram	1 gram	3 grams
Fiber	0 grams	0 grams	0 grams
Sugar	1 gram	less than 1 gram	2 grams
Sodium	150 mg	170 mg	150 mg

Nutrition facts for popular brands of spinach dip

The next chart reveals the nutrient facts for around 2 tablespoons (28–32 grams) of common store-bought spinach dips

	Tostitos Creamy Spinach Dip	Cedar's Spinach Dip	TGI Friday's Frozen Spinach Artichoke Dip
Calories	50	50	30
Protein	1 gram	1 gram	2 grams
Total fat	4 grams	4 grams	2 grams
Saturated fat	0 grams	1 gram	1 gram
Carbs	2 grams	3 grams	2 grams
Fiber	1 gram	0 grams	0 grams
Sugar	1 gram	2 grams	1 gram
Sodium	190 mg	140 mg	135 mg

SUMMARY

Spinach dip typically contains 30–100 calories per 2-tablespoon (30-gram) serving. It's generally low in fiber and moderate to high in fat.

Health benefits of spinach dip

Spinach dip tends to be more of an indulgent, occasional treat — but depending how you make it, it may offer some health benefits.

May boost your vegetable intake

The amount of spinach in spinach dip varies significantly from one brand to another, as well as one recipe to the next.

If you make it yourself, you can include more spinach and even other vegetables like artichokes, which can boost your veggie — and nutrient — intake.

Spinach (both fresh and frozen) is a good source of fiber, several B vitamins, and vitamins A, C, E, K. It also contains minerals like iron, magnesium, calcium, manganese, potassium, and copper.

If you add artichokes, you'll get <u>extra fiber</u>, folate, and vitamins C and K.

Serving this dip with veggie sticks made from carrots, cucumbers, bell peppers, broccoli, celery, or zucchini may also help you meet the U.S. Department of Agriculture's (USDA's) recommended 2–3 cups (120–200 grams) of vegetables per day.

Since only 9% of Americans meet this guidance, finding ways to eat more vegetables is essential for overall health.

May serve as a filling snack

Spinach dip made with Greek yogurt and vegetable oil-based mayonnaise may contribute protein and healthy fats to your diet, both of which can help you feel full.

When paired with either high fiber veggies or fiber-rich whole grain crackers or bread, it may be even more filling.

Choosing snacks that are enjoyable and filling may help you eat less overall and maintain a healthy weight. However, it can be easy to overeat snacks, so be sure to eat mindfully and stop when you're full.

SUMMARY

Versions of spinach dip made with plenty of veggies and sources of protein like Greek yogurt may boost your nutrient intake and help you stay full.

Potential downsides of spinach dip

Some spinach dips provide very few nutrients and may contribute excess calories, saturated fat, and sodium to your diet.

May provide saturated fat

Depending on the recipe or product, spinach dip may be high in saturated fat — especially if it's made with full fat cream cheese or other cheeses.

For example, 1/4 cup (60 grams) of store-bought spinach dip made with parmesan and cream cheese contains 6 grams of saturated fat.

While some studies suggest that too much saturated fat may raise cholesterol and your risk of heart disease and diabetes, other research has found no link between saturated fat intake — especially from dairy foods — and increased risk of heart disease.

That said, the USDA recommends keeping saturated fat intake to less than 10% of total calories, or about 22 grams for someone eating 2,000 calories per day.

The American Heart Association (AHA) has an even lower threshold of less than 6% of calories, or 13 grams per day for a 2,000 calorie diet.

If you decide to watch your saturated fat intake, choose a yogurt-based spinach dip that's light on the cheese — or skips it altogether.

May be calorie dense

Most spinach dips range from 50–100 calories per 2-tablespoon (30–gram) serving. Yet, it's reasonable to assume that most people eat more than this amount of dip at one sitting. A more realistic serving size is probably 1/4 cup (60 grams), which packs 100–200 calories.

When paired with chips, bread, or crackers, spinach dip may easily become high in calories.

Studies indicate that eating high calorie snacks may lead you to eat more than necessary in a day, which may lead to weight gain

To keep calories in check, choose yogurt-based spinach dip, serve with vegetables instead of chips, and limit yourself to small portions.

May be paired with refined carbs

Spinach dip is often served with chips, crackers, pita bread, or other white bread for dipping.

If eaten in excess, refined carbs like these are linked to an increased risk of type 2 diabetes and heart disease. They may also lead to blood sugar spikes, which in turn cause a crash in energy levels.

Choosing whole grain carbs like whole grain crackers or whole wheat pita for dipping instead of refined carbs may reduce this snack's effect on your blood sugar.

May be high in sodium

Spinach dip is often high in sodium, especially in large amounts or if served with salty chips or crackers.

The AHA recommends that you keep sodium intake to less than 2,300 mg per day, and less than 1,500 mg per day if you have a high risk of heart disease.

Research indicates that excess sodium may contribute to elevated blood pressure and heart disease risk.

If you're watching your sodium intake, you may want to make your own spinach dip and limit added salt and cheese, which can be high in sodium.

SUMMARY

Spinach dip is often high in sodium, paired with refined carbs, and calorie dense. For some individuals, its saturated fat content may also be worth noting. Overall, it's worth keeping your intake in moderation.

Store-bought vs. homemade spinach dip

The health effects of both store-bought and homemade dips differ depending on the ingredients. Notably, you have much more control over the ingredients — and therefore the nutritional value — if you make it yourself.

Ultimately, choosing one or the other depends on your nutrition needs, desire to cook, how you want to serve it (hot or cold), and how much time you have.

Distinctions of store-bought dips

Store-bought dips are often higher in sodium because salt is used not only as a flavoring but also as a preservative, extending the product's shelf-life.

Spinach dip packets, which include seasonings for you to mix into homemade dip, tend to be high in sodium as well.

Plus, pre-made dips more likely contain added sugar, food stabilizers, and other additives.

Distinctions of homemade dips

Depending on the recipe, ingredients vary widely for homemade spinach dips.

More indulgent dips include cream cheese, mayonnaise, and cheeses like parmesan or mozzarella whereas lighter options are made with yogurt, more vegetables, and little or no cheese.

Homemade spinach dips are also sometimes served warm, which can be a nice treat — especially at a party.

SUMMARY

Store-bought spinach dips tend to have more preservatives and salt than homemade versions, while homemade versions are sometimes served warm and give you more control over the ingredients.

Tips for making healthy homemade spinach tip

Here are a few easy tips for making nutritious spinach dip at home.

Load up on the veggies

The more spinach you add to your dip, the more nutritious it will be. You can also add other veggies like:

- onions
- bell peppers
- artichokes
- water chestnuts
- sun dried tomatoes
- roasted mushrooms

Serve with veggie sticks instead of crackers

Furthermore, you can serve your dip with sliced veggies rather than crackers or chips. Almost any fresh vegetable works great with spinach dip, but here are a few ideas:

- baby carrots or sliced carrots
- sliced bell peppers
- cherry tomatoes
- celery sticks
- zucchini slices
- broccoli or cauliflower florets

Dehydrated vegetables or baked veggie chips are also good dipping options.

Use plain Greek yogurt

Plain Greek yogurt adds protein to your dip, which can make it more filling. While low fat Greek yogurt may reduce the saturated fat content of the dip, full fat Greek yogurt is creamier, creating a more satisfying texture and flavor.

You can use Greek yogurt in place of some or all of the mayonnaise and cream cheese in your recipe. You may still want to use small amounts of mayo, parmesan, or mozzarella for flavor and texture.

Limit the cheese, and choose healthy types

Cheese is a great way to flavor your spinach dip, but you may want to limit the total amount to keep calories, saturated fat, and sodium in check.

You may also want to choose certain types over others. Good options include:

- **Parmesan.** This cheese is a good source of calcium and protein. Although it's higher in sodium than some other cheeses, a little goes a long way.

- **Cheddar.** This popular orange cheese contains calcium, some protein, and small amounts of vitamin K2, which has been shown to support bone and heart health.

- **Mozzarella.** This soft, white cheese is commonly used in spinach dip. It's lower in sodium and calories than many cheeses and may even contain probiotics, which boost your gut health.

On the other hand, cream cheese tends to be high in calories. Consider cutting back on it or replacing it with Greek yogurt or cottage cheese.

Watch the added salt

Excess sodium and sugar may increase your risk of heart disease and type 2 diabetes.

Sodium is found in mayonnaise, cheese, and cream cheese — three common ingredients in spinach dips. Many recipes also call for additional salt.

If you already follow a low sodium diet, the salt in spinach dip may not be a concern. However, to be on the safe side, you may want to:

- Limit the total amount of salt in your recipe.

- Check the nutrient info for store-bought dips.

- Use veggie sticks for dipping instead of salty chips or crackers.

- Use fresh or dried herbs as seasoning instead of salt.

Serve with healthy accompaniments

If you choose to serve your veggie dip with crackers or chips, it's best to choose healthy options made from whole grains. Options include:

- veggie chips like kale, carrot, or beet chips

- whole grain pita bread, toasted

- whole grain crackers

SUMMARY

To make healthy spinach dip, load up on the veggies, choose small amounts of healthy cheese, watch the salt, and serve with veggie sticks or whole grain crackers.

The bottom line

The health effects of spinach dip depend entirely on how it's made and what you serve it with.

Some recipes or pre-made dips contain a lot of sodium and calories, which you may want to limit.

However, you can make spinach dip a healthy snack or appetizer by using Greek yogurt, limiting added cheese, and serving it with vegetables or whole grain crackers for dipping.

Plus, spinach dip isn't an everyday food for most people, so even the more indulgent recipes can be part of a healthy diet. Try to keep portion sizes moderate — about 1/4 cup (60 grams).

If you enjoy it most when it's made with mayonnaise, cream cheese, and cheese, it's OK to enjoy it on occasion.

10 Delicious Diabetic-Friendly Smoothies

Overview

Having diabetes doesn't mean you need to deny yourself all the foods you love, but you do want to make healthier food choices. One good choice is to eat a lot of fruits and vegetables, which are heavy in nutrition but light in calories.

Some fruits and vegetables are better for managing your diabetes than others. Look for produce that's low on the glycemic index and load, meaning it won't spike your blood sugar.

It's also important to get plenty of calcium- and probiotic-rich dairy foods to fortify your bones and provide good gut bacteria. Good sources are low-fat milk, kefir, and Greek yogurt.

These foods are essential to any diabetes diet, yet you don't need to eat them with a fork or even a spoon. You can pack a lot of nutrition into one smoothie and get a delicious treat. As long as you stick with healthy ingredients and don't add extra sweeteners, you can enjoy these treats on a regular basis.

Just remember when you do blend fruit into your smoothies to count them as part of your daily fruit allowance so you don't overdo it on carbohydrates. Even natural sugar can drive up your blood sugar if you eat too much of it.

Here are 10 diabetes-friendly smoothie ideas to get you started.

Superfood smoothie

This smoothie has it all — antioxidant-rich berries, healthy fat from the avocado, greens, and protein. Just be careful when buying berry yogurt that you choose a brand that's low in sugar, such as Siggi, or stevia-sweetened. Or opt for unsweetened yogurt.

This recipe has 404 calories, so use it as a meal replacement instead of a snack.

Lower-carb strawberry smoothie

This smoothie's creator has diabetes and discovered this recipe after some careful experimentation.

Not only does it taste great, but also it won't wreak havoc on your blood sugar. The soymilk and Greek yogurt make it smooth and creamy without adding much extra sugar. You can even bump up the fiber more with a tablespoon of chia seeds.

Berry blast smoothie

The berry base of this smoothie makes it sweet, yet it's still low on the glycemic index. If your berries are tart, the coconut milk and mango will add some natural sweetness. You'll also get a healthy dose of omega-3 fatty acids from the flax.

This recipe makes two smoothies.

Peach smoothie

This peach smoothie makes for the perfect afternoon refresher. It's simple to make with only five ingredients. Plus, it's loaded with calcium and is light enough that it won't weigh you down.

Add 1 tablespoon of chia seeds and keep the peel on the peach for more fiber. More fiber is helpful in this smoothie because this recipe calls for 4 ounces of sweetened yogurt, which has the potential to raise your blood sugar.

Joann's green smoothie

This smoothie sneaks in a green vegetable, spinach, but camouflages it with fresh berries and chocolate powder. Choose stevia- or erythritol-sweetened protein powder to avoid artificial sweeteners. Chia seeds and pumpkin seeds add a rich texture, fiber, and omega-3 fatty acids.

The greenie green smoothie

If you're having trouble meeting your daily green requirements but aren't a big fan of salads, why not drink your veggies? This take on the increasingly popular green smoothie uses nutrient-dense kale or spinach balanced with tart apple and pear. Lime juice and mint complement the blend, adding a burst of flavor and freshness.

Skip the agave nectar, which may have negative effects on your metabolism.

Snickers smoothie

Are you craving the chocolate-peanut taste of your favorite candy bar, but don't want to send your blood sugar soaring? Get the same flavors without the spike by whipping up this candy-inspired smoothie. For less artificial sweetener, swap the 1 tablespoon of sugar-free caramel syrup for 1 teaspoon of caramel extract.

This smoothie is high in protein and calcium.

Chia seed, coconut, and spinach smoothie

This rich and creamy smoothie contains only 5 grams of carbohydrates. To keep the carbs down, use unsweetened light coconut milk. For added sweetness, the author recommends adding a few dashes of powdered Stevia.

Diabetic oatmeal breakfast smoothie

What better way to start your day than with some hearty, fiber-dense whole grains, plus potassium and vitamin C? The uncooked oats also provide resistant starch, which is an excellent source of fuel for gut bacteria and can improve insulin levels.

This breakfast smoothie packs a lot of nutrition into one glass. Here are a few tips to make this smoothie work better for your blood sugar:

- Choose smaller bananas and don't forget to add those carbs to your daily count so you don't go over your allotment.

- Turn this recipe into four servings rather than two.

- Use unsweetened almond or soymilk instead of skim milk to further reduce the carbs.

Berry delicious nutty milkshake

Nuts are an important component of any healthy eating plan, and this recipe combines some of the most nutritious varieties, almonds and walnuts. Plus, you get greens from the kale, calcium from the milk, and antioxidants from the strawberries. All this for only 45 grams of carbohydrate!

Spinach Extract: An Effective Weight Loss Supplement?

People who want to lose weight often turn to supplements, hoping for an easy solution. However, the effects of most supplements are usually disappointing.

One weight loss supplement that entered the market recently is called spinach extract. It's claimed to cause weight loss by reducing appetite and cravings.

This article provides a detailed review of spinach extract and its weight loss effects.

What Is Spinach Extract?

Spinach extract is a weight loss supplement made from spinach leaves.

It is also known by the brand name Appethyl, which is owned by the Swedish company Greenleaf Medical AB.

Spinach extract is a green powder that can be mixed with water or smoothies. It's also sold in other forms, including capsules and snack bars.

The powder consists of concentrated spinach leaf thylakoids, which are microscopic structures found inside the chloroplasts of green plant cells.

The role of the thylakoids is to harvest sunlight — a process known as photosynthesis — which provides plants with the energy they need to produce carbs.

Thylakoids are composed of about 70% proteins, antioxidants, and chlorophyll, while the other 30% mostly consists of fat.

Thylakoids are not unique to spinach leaves. In fact, they're found in the leaves of all green plants — and similar supplements could be made from those plants as well.

Note that other supplements may also be called spinach extract, but this article only refers to the type of thylakoid concentrate found in Appethyl.

SUMMARY

Spinach extract — also known as Appethyl — is a weight loss supplement. It contains thylakoids, which consist mostly of proteins, antioxidants, and chlorophyll.

How Does It Work?

Thylakoids from spinach extract suppress the activity of lipase, an enzyme that digests fat.

This helps delay fat digestion, which increases your levels of appetite-reducing hormones like glucagon-like peptide-1 (GLP-1). It also reduces levels of ghrelin, the hunger hormone.

Unlike pharmaceutical weight loss drugs like orlistat, thylakoids cause a temporary delay in fat digestion but don't prevent it completely.

As a result, spinach extract doesn't have the unpleasant side effects of other lipase-inhibiting drugs, such as fatty stools and stomach cramps.

It's not entirely clear what part of the thylakoids is responsible for these effects, but they may be caused by certain proteins or fats called galactolipids.

SUMMARY

Spinach extract promotes weight loss by delaying fat digestion, temporarily reducing appetite, and causing you to eat less.

Can It Help You Lose Weight?

Animal studies show that taking thylakoid-rich spinach extract may reduce body fat and weight.

Studies in overweight adults indicate that adding 3.7–5 grams of spinach extract to a meal reduces appetite for several hours.

By suppressing appetite, spinach extract may lead to weight loss if taken regularly over a few months.

One study in overweight women found that consuming 5 grams of spinach extract every day as part of a 3-month weight loss program resulted in 43% greater weight loss than a placebo.

Body mass index (BMI), fat mass, and lean mass decreased as well, but differences across groups were insignificant.

Plus, it should be noted that some of the researchers involved in this study had financial ties to the company that developed the supplement.

Therefore, the findings need to be confirmed by an independent research group.

SUMMARY

Studies show that taking spinach extract supplements for a few months may cause weight loss. However, due to a potential conflict of interest, further studies are needed.

May Fight Cravings

Spinach extract may suppress your brain's food reward system, reducing cravings.

When overweight women consumed 5 grams of spinach extract per day, cravings for sweets and chocolate decreased by 95% and 87%, respectively.

Another study in women suggests that 5 grams of spinach extract reduces cravings for snack foods, including those that are salty, sweet, and fatty. However, no effects on calorie intake at a later buffet were observed.

The reduction in cravings may be because spinach extract promotes the release of glucagon-like peptide-1 (GLP-1), which acts on your food reward system.

SUMMARY

Spinach extract may suppress your brain's food reward system, temporarily reducing cravings. Over time, this contributes to weight loss.

Safety and Side Effects

Spinach extract appears to be without serious side effects.

In healthy people, it may temporarily reduce insulin levels and increase blood sugar.

Still, it does not seem to have long-term effects on blood sugar control.

Nonetheless, further studies are needed to assess the safety of spinach extract for people with type 2 diabetes.

SUMMARY

Spinach extract may reduce insulin levels temporarily. Otherwise, its use appears to be safe and without side effects.

Dosage and How to Use

An effective dose of spinach extract is about 4–5 grams when taken with a meal. However, you may need to take it for a few months before you see any effects on your weight.

Since spinach extract delays fat digestion and reduces appetite for a few hours, it's of greater use when taken before a meal that contains fat.

You shouldn't expect to see any significant benefits from the supplement alone. As with all weight loss supplements, you also need to make some healthy lifestyle changes.

SUMMARY

Spinach extract is of most use when taken with meals that contain fat. An effective dose is 4–5 grams per day.

The Bottom Line

Evidence suggests that spinach extract may be an effective weight loss supplement.

By delaying fat digestion, it temporarily reduces appetite and cravings. When combined with other lifestyle modifications, this may lead to significant weight loss.

However, many of the scientists studying spinach extract have industry ties. Further studies by independent research groups would strengthen the evidence.

Table of Contents

Smoothies for Diabetics Introduction

Recipes have only ingredients listed and instructions how to blend a perfect smoothie are given here as a short introduction:

Put the liquid in first. Surrounded by tea or yogurt, the blender blades can move freely. Next, add chunks of fruits or vegetables. Leafy greens are going into the pitcher last. Preferred liquid is green tea, but you can use almond or coconut milk or herbal tea.

Start slow. If your blender has speeds, start it on low to break up big pieces of fruit. Continue blending until you get a puree. If your blender can pulse, pulse a few times before switching to a puree mode. Once you have your liquid and fruit pureed, start adding greens, very slowly. Wait until previous batch of greens has been completely blended. I use blenders because they're sturdy and offer 7 year warranty. That was definitely the best investment in my health.

Thicken? Added too much tea or coconut milk? Thicken your smoothie by adding ice cubes, flax meal, chia seeds or oatmeal. Once you get used to various tastes of smoothies, add any seaweed, spirulina, chlorella powder or ginger for additional kick. Experiment with any Superfoods in powder form at this point. Think of adding any nut butter or sesame paste too or some Superfoods oils.

Rotate! Rotate your greens; don't always drink the same smoothie! At the beginning try 2 different greens every week and later introduce third and fourth one weekly. And keep rotating them. Don't use spinach and kale all the time. Try beets greens, they have a pinch of pink in them and that add great color to your smoothie. Here is the list of leafy green for you to try: spinach, kale, dandelion, chards, beet leaves, arugula, lettuce, collard greens, bok choy, cabbage, cilantro, parsley.

Flavor! Flavor smoothies with ground vanilla bean, cinnamon, ½ tsp. of lucuma powder, nutmeg, cloves, almond butter, cayenne pepper, ginger or just about any seeds or chopped nuts combination.

Not only are green smoothies high in nutrients, vitamins and fiber, they can also make any vegetable you probably don't like (be it kale, spinach or broccoli) taste great. The secret behind blending the perfect smoothie is using sweet fruits or nuts or seeds to give your drink a unique taste.

There's a reason kale and spinach seem to be the main ingredients in almost every green smoothie. Not only do they give smoothies their verdant color, they are also packed with calcium, protein and iron.

Although blending alone increases the accessibility of carotenoids, since the presence of fats is known to increase carotenoid absorption from leafy greens, it is possible that coconut oil, nuts and seeds in a smoothie could increase absorption further.

• Wash fruits and veggies

• Pluck leaves and stems from berries

• Core apples (optional)

• Peel orange, lemon, lime, grapefruit, kiwi, beet, pomegranate, ginger, dragon fruit and banana

• Peel and take the seeds out of papaya

• Remove seeds from peppers, apricots, peaches, cherries, plums and prunes

• Mangos, melons and avocados should be peeled, and inner seed taken out

• Watermelons should have their outer rind removed.

• Scoop out the flesh from passion fruit

• Cut fruits and veggies in 2-inch slices

Spinach Berries Smoothie

- ½ cup almond milk
- ½ cup water
- 1 carrot
- 1 cup spinach
- 1 cup frozen raspberries
- 1 tablespoon seeds
- 1 tablespoon fresh mint
- ½ teaspoon powder

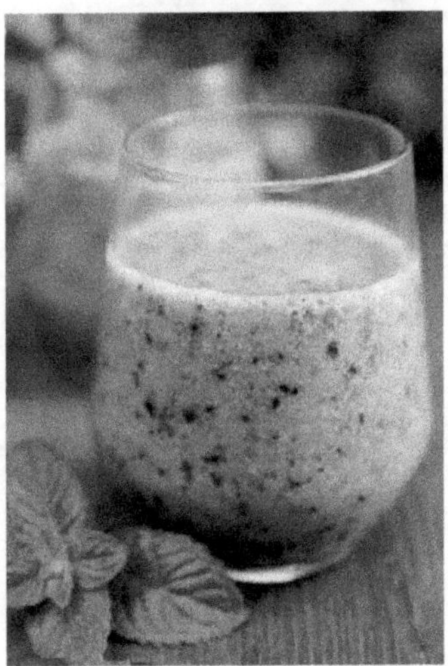

Apricots & Carrots Smoothie

4 apricots

1 apple

1 cup red spinach

2 carrots

1 cup water

1 tbsp.

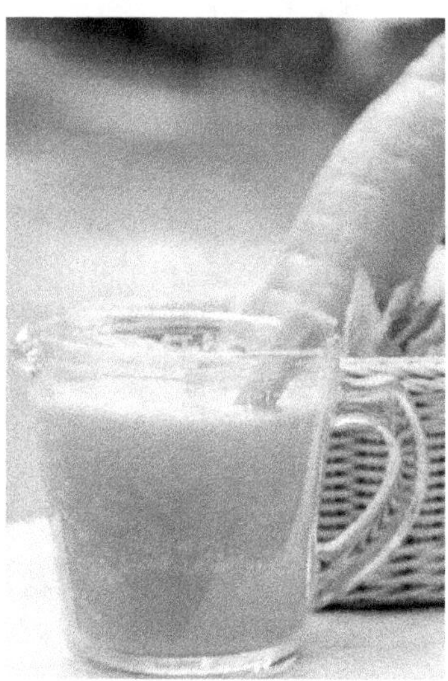

Radicchio Cranberry Smoothie

- 1 cup fresh Cranberries
- 1 apple
- ½ cup Red Spinach
- ½ Avocado
- 1/2 cup chopped Radicchio
- 1 tbsp.
- 1 cup crushed ice

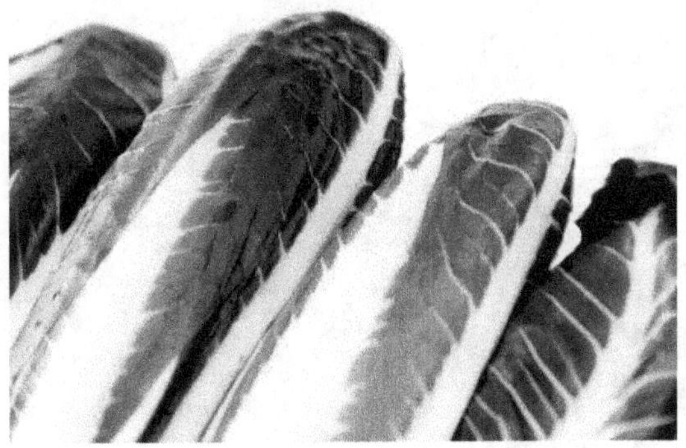

Papaya Red Spinach Smoothie

- 1 cup chopped Papaya

- 1 banana

- 1 cup red spinach

- 1 cup crushed ice

- 1 tablespoon

- Top with 1 tablespoon dried chokecherries

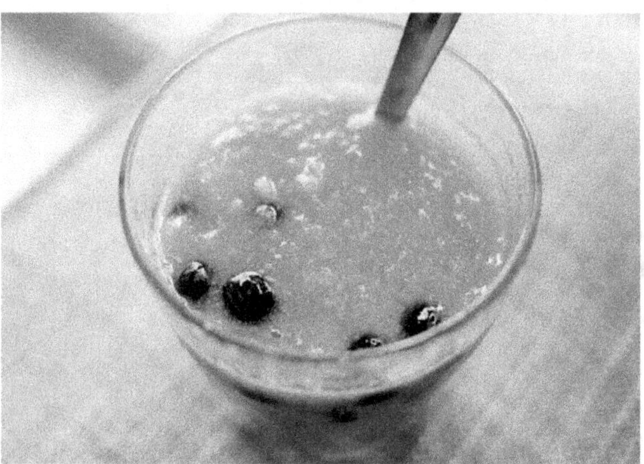

Blueberry Avocado Smoothie

- 1/2 avocado

- 1 cup spinach

- 1 cup blueberries, frozen

- 1 tsp. oil

- 3/4 cup water

- 1 cup crushed ice

- Top with Cranberries

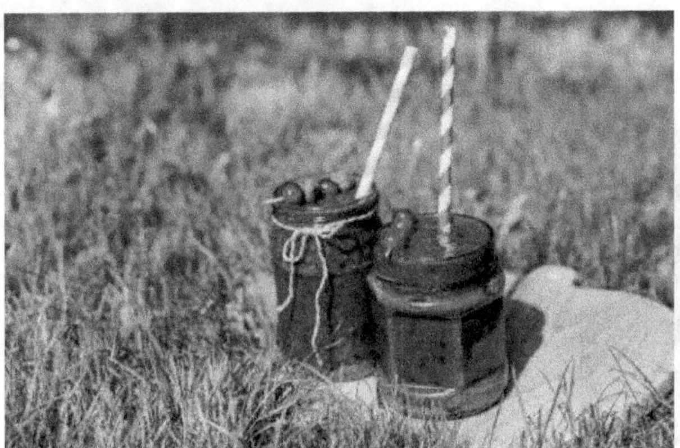

Beet Spinach Smoothie

- 1 large beet

- 1 apple

- 1 blood orange

- ½ cup frozen blackberries

- 1 cup spinach

- ½ cup crushed ice

- ½ cup water

- 1 tbsp. Seeds

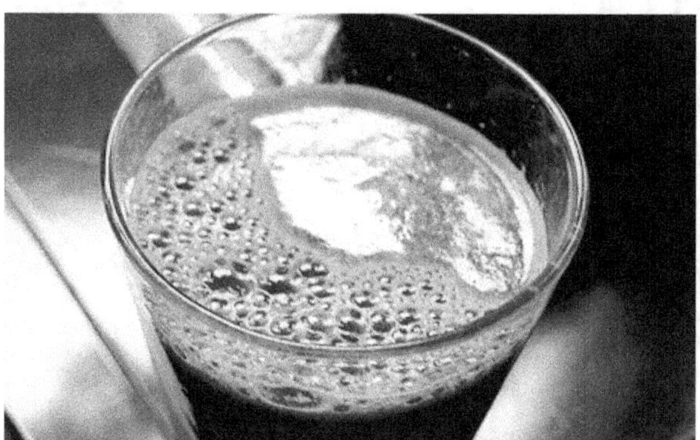

Blueberry Kefir & Spinach Smoothie

- 1 cup blueberries

- 1 cup chopped Cantaloupe

- 1 cup Spinach

- 1 cup Kefir

- 1 tbsp. seeds

- ½ tsp. Cinnamon

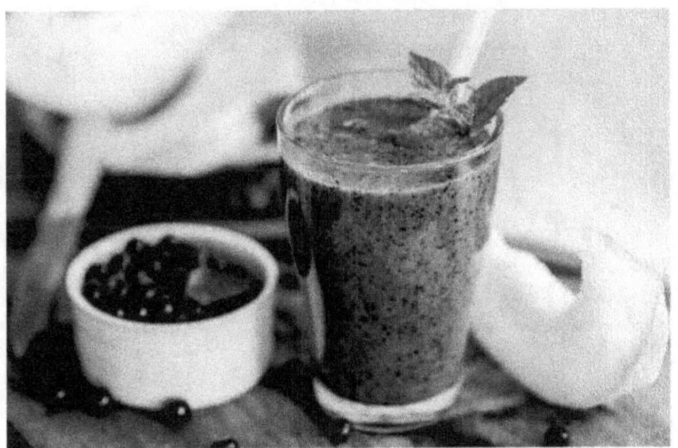

Spinach Smoothie

- 1 cup Dandelion greens

- 1 cup Spinach

- ½ cup tahini

- 1 Red Radish

- 1 tbsp. seeds

- 1 cup lavender tea

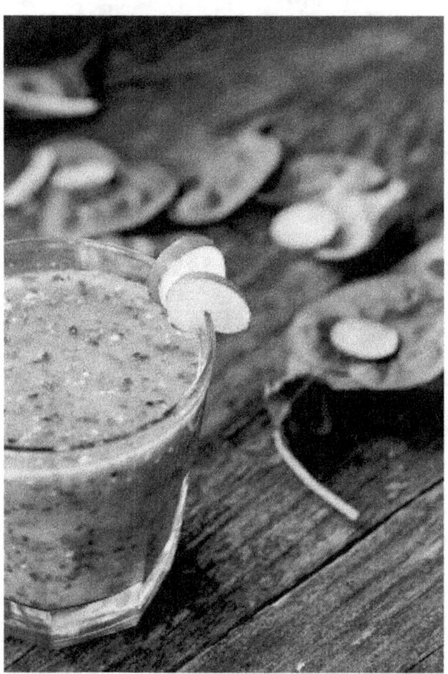

Broccoli Apple Smoothie

- 1 Apple

- 1 cup Broccoli

- 1 tbsp. Cilantro

- 1 Celery stalk

- 1 cup crushed ice

- 1 tbsp. crushed Seaweed

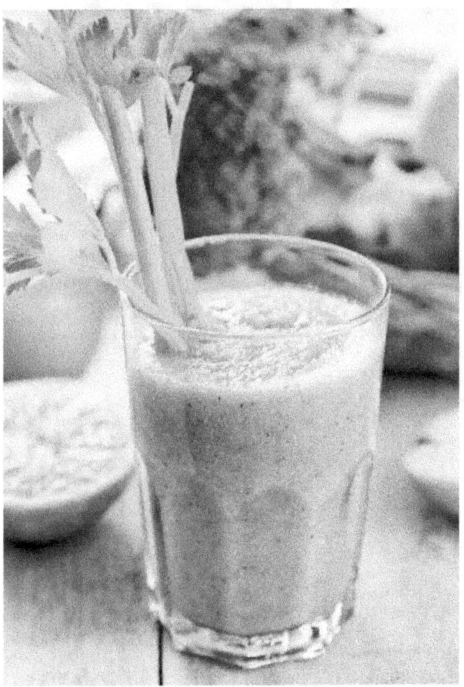

Salad Smoothie

- 1 cup spinach

- ½ cucumber

- 1/2 small onion

- 2 tablespoons Parsley

- 2 tablespoons lemon juice

- 1 cup crushed ice

- 1 tbsp. olive oil

- ¼ cup Wheatgrass

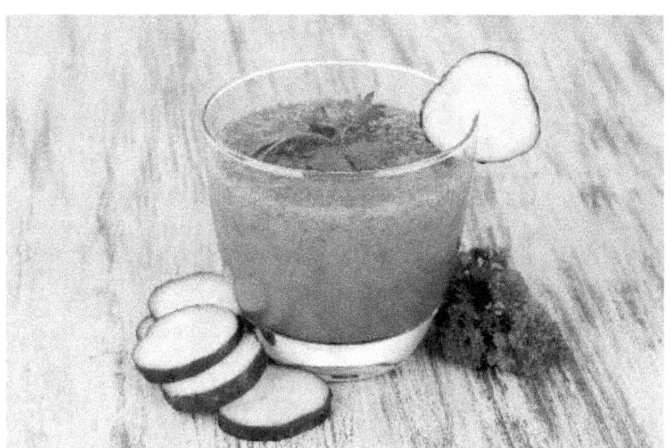

Cacao Spinach Smoothie

- 2 cups spinach

- 1 cup blueberries, frozen

- 1 tablespoons dark cocoa powder

- ½ cup unsweetened almond milk

- 1/2 cup crushed ice

- 1/2 tsp powder

- 1 tbsp. powder

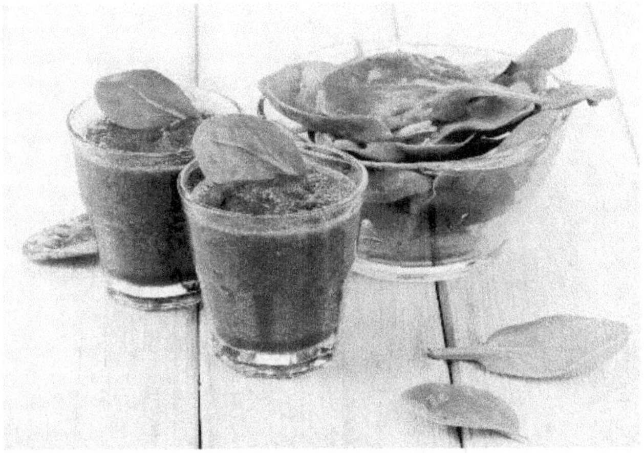

Flax Almond Butter Smoothie

- ½ cup plain yogurt
- 2 tablespoons almond butter
- 2 cups spinach
- 1 banana, frozen
- 3 strawberries
- 1/2 cup crushed ice
- 1 teaspoon seed

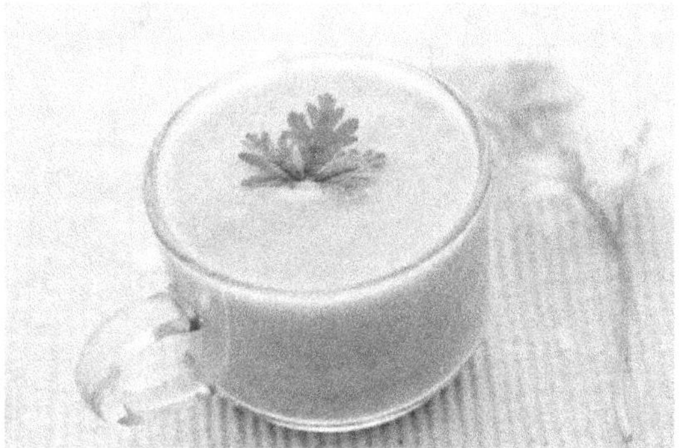

Banana Spinach Raspberry Smoothie

- 1 cup Spinach
- 2 Bananas
- 2
- ½ cup Raspberries
- 1 tbsp. Ground seeds
- 1 cup crushed ice
- 1 tbsp. Cilantro

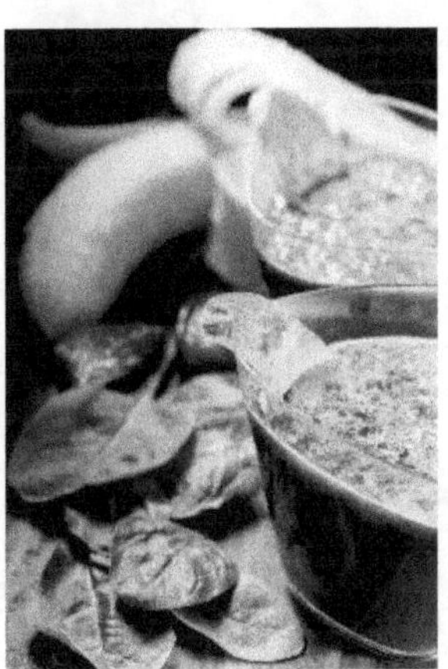

Spinach Celery Parsley Smoothie

- 1 cup Spinach

- 1 Peach

- 1 avocado

- 2 stalks Celery

- 1 Lime

- 1 tbsp. seeds

- 1 cup crushed ice

- 1 tbsp. Parsley

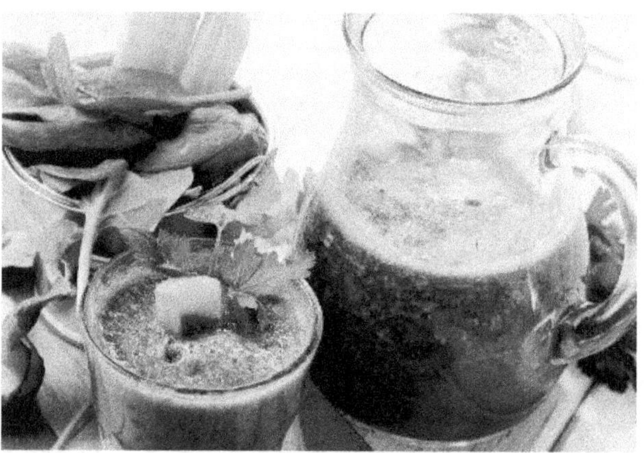

Spinach Cucumber Celery Carrot Smoothie

- 1 cup Spinach
- 2 Carrots
- 1 Cucumber
- 2 stalks Celery
- 1 Tbsp. powder
- 1 tbsp. Parsley
- 1 cup crushed ice

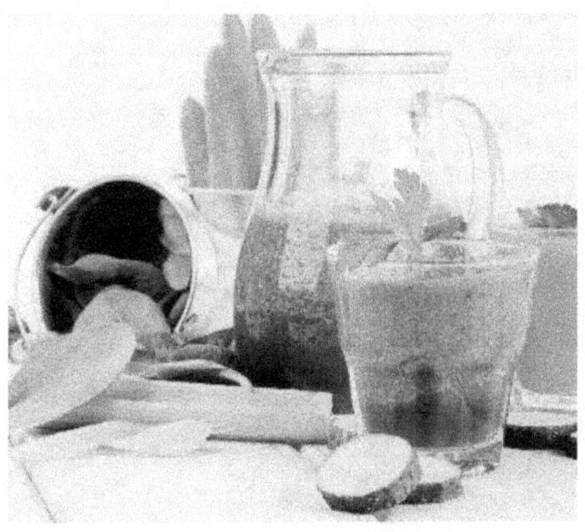

Kiwi Spinach Smoothie

- 1 cup spinach

- 2 Apples

- 1/2 avocado

- 2 kiwis

- 1 tbsp.

- 1 cup crushed ice

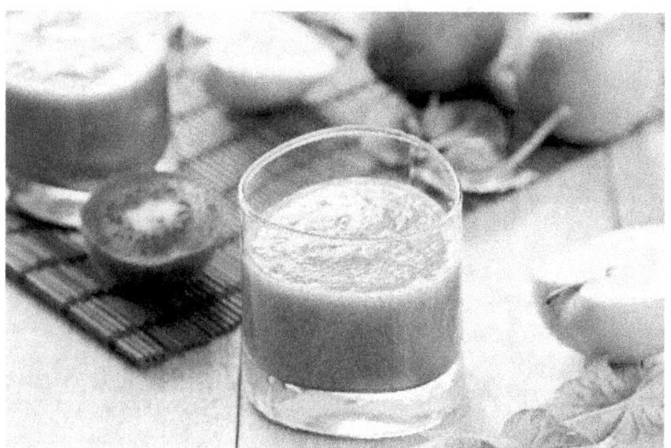

Flax Kiwi Spinach Smoothie

- 1 cup Spinach

- 1 Apple

- 1 banana

- 1 stalk Celery

- 2 Kiwis

- 3 tbsp. ground seeds

- 1 cup crushed ice

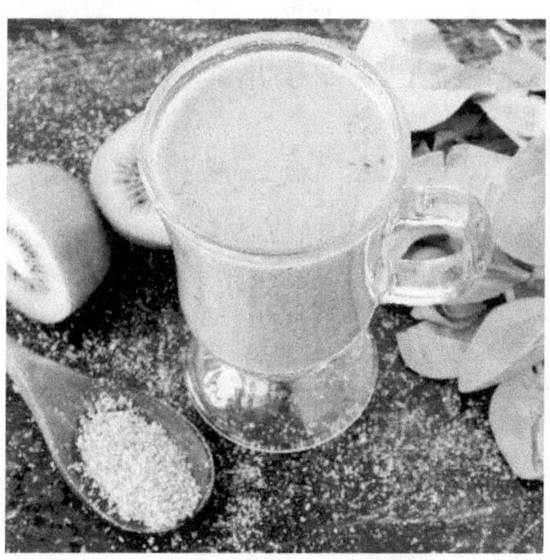

Leaf Lettuce Apples Spinach Smoothie

- 1/2 cup Spinach

- 2 Apples

- 2 Tbsp. almond butter

- 1 cup Leaf Lettuce

- 1/2 Lemon

- 1 tbsp.

- 1 cup crushed ice

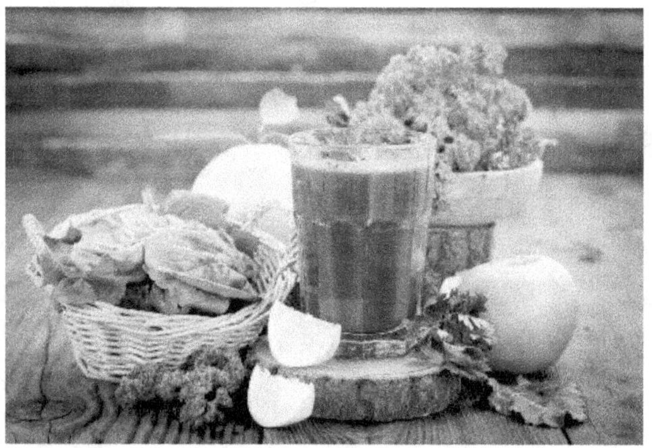

Dandelion Banana Smoothie

- 1/2 cup Dandelion leaves

- 1/2 cup spinach leaves

- 2 Bananas

- 3/4 avocado

- 1 Orange

- 1 tbsp.

- 1 cup crushed ice

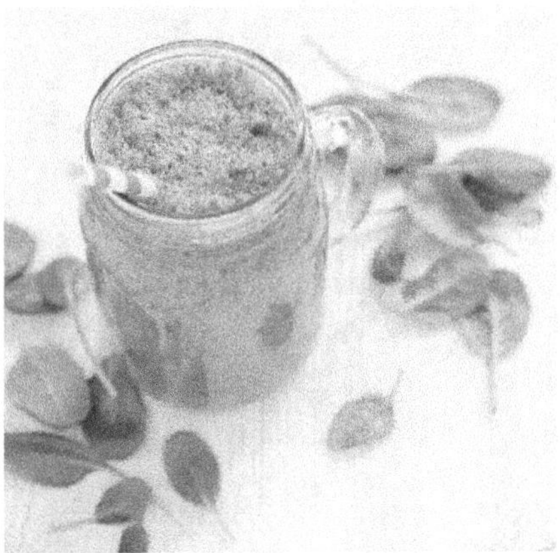

Chia Apples Spinach Smoothie

- 1 cup Spinach or mustard greens

- 2 Apples

- 2 tbsp. Tahini

- 3 tbsp. seeds

- 1 cup crushed ice

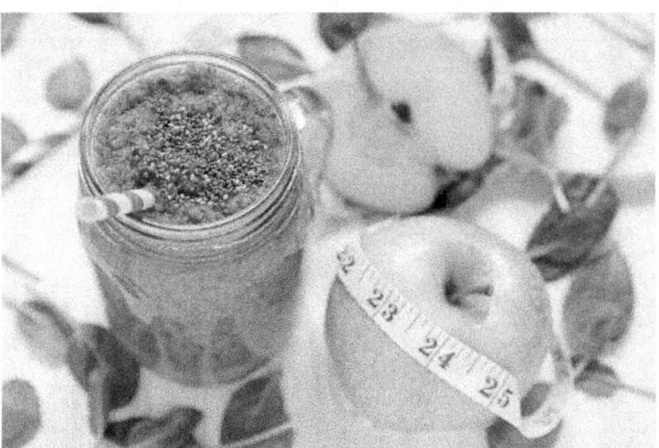

Dandelion Apples Smoothie

- 1/2 cup Dandelion leaves

- 1/2 cup spinach leaves

- 1 orange

- 3/4 avocado

- 1 stalk Celery or 1 broccoli floret

- 1 tsp. chopped fresh ginger

- 1 cup crushed ice

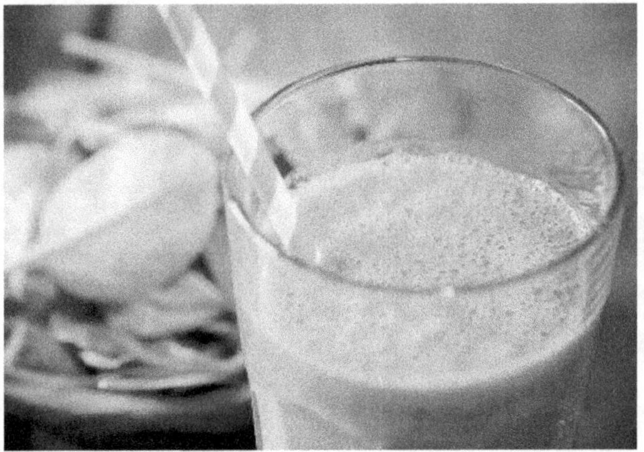

Chia, Spinach & Kiwi Smoothie

- 1 cup Spinach leaves
- 3 kiwis
- 1 Tbsp. tahini
- 1 3 Tbsp. Chia seeds
- 1 cup crushed ice

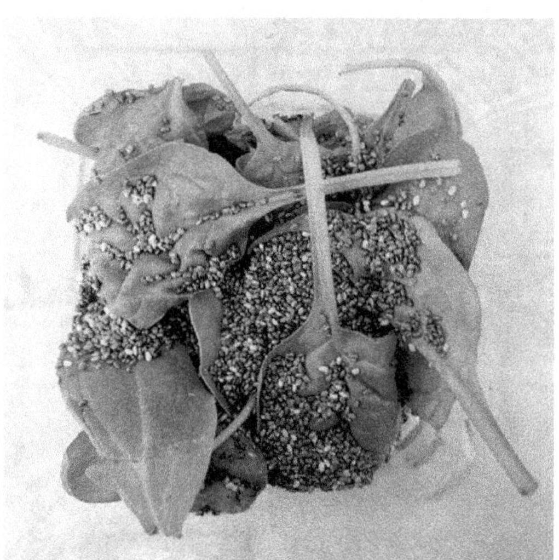

Yellow Pumpkin, Peach & Spinach Smoothie

- 1 cup Spinach leaves

- 1 cup cooked yellow pumpkin

- 1 cup cubed peach

- 3/4 avocado

- a pinch of nutmeg and cinnamon

- 1 tbsp. lucuma

- 1 cup crushed ice

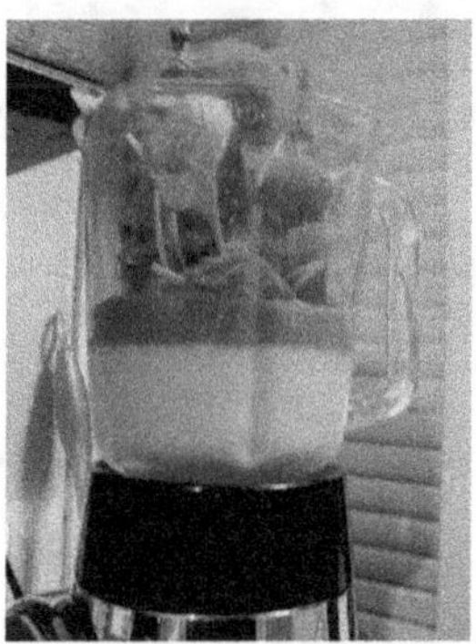

Papaya, Peach & Spinach Smoothie

- 1 cup Spinach leaves

- 1 cup cubed papaya

- 3/4 avocado

- 1 cup cubed peach

- 1 cup crushed ice

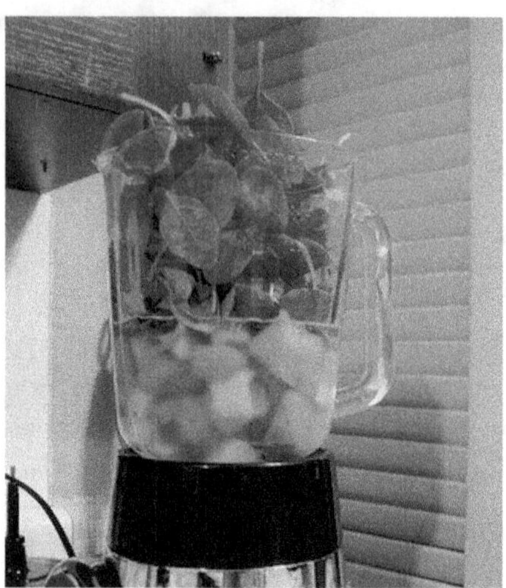

Spinach Celery Apples Smoothie

- 1 cup spinach
- 2 Apples
- 2 Tbsp. almond butter
- 1 tbsp. Chia seeds
- 1 cup crushed ice

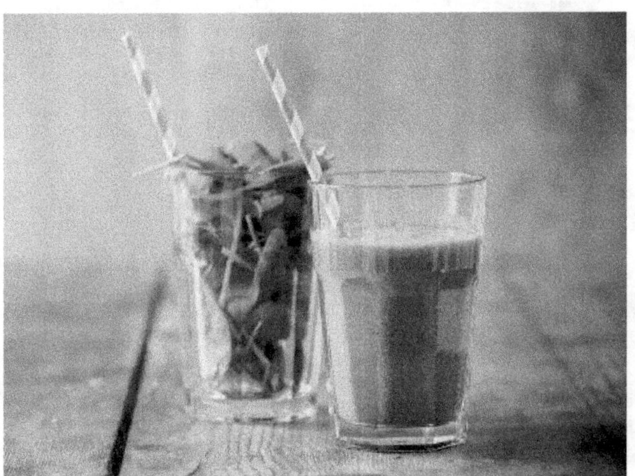

Papaya Spinach Smoothie

- 1 banana

- 1 cup spinach

- 1 cup chopped papaya

- 1 cup crushed ice

- 1 tbsp. seeds

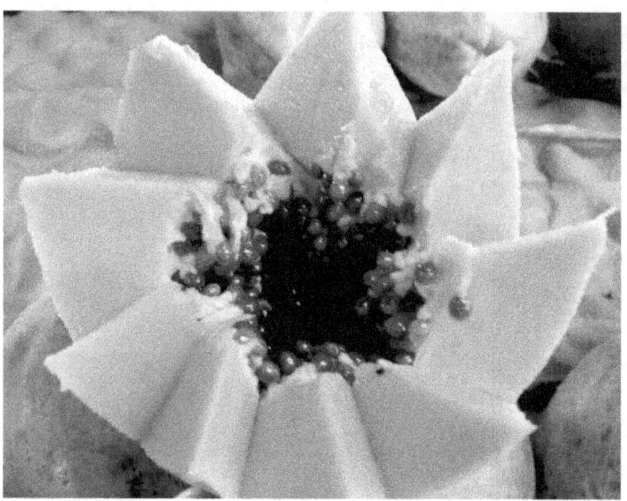

Kefir Blueberry Mixed Greens Smoothie

- 1 cup Kefir

- 1 cup blueberries

- 1 cup mixed greens (spinach included)

- 1 cup crushed ice

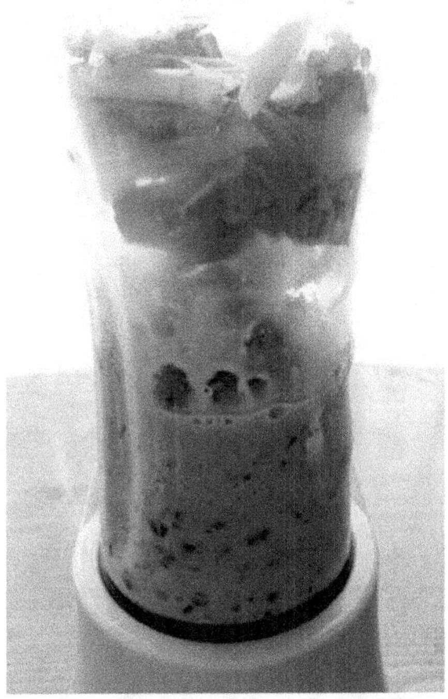

Banana Orange Mixed Greens Smoothie

- 1 Orange
- 1 banana
- 1 cup mixed greens (spinach included)
- 1/2 cup blackberries
- 1 cup crushed ice

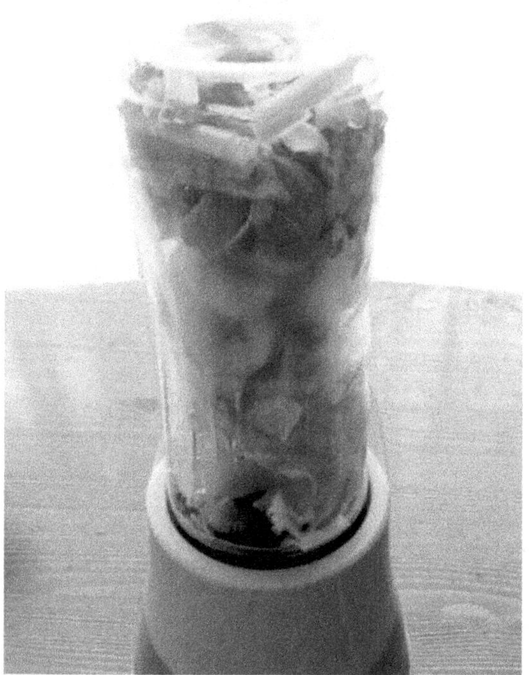

Celery Spinach Avocado Smoothie

- 1 cup celery

- 1 avocado

- 1 cup spinach

- 1 cup crushed ice

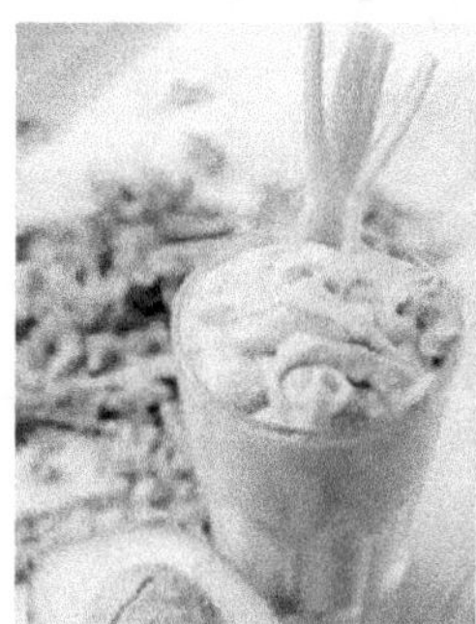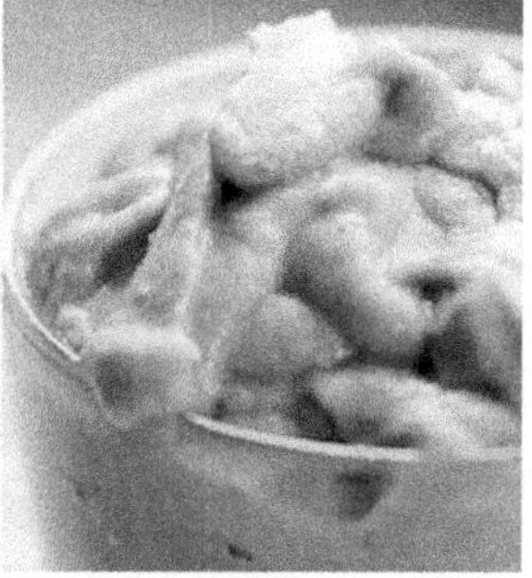

Cucumber Watermelon Strawberries Spinach Smoothie

- 1 Cucumber
- 1 cup watermelon
- 1 cup Spinach
- 1 cup strawberries
- 1 cup crushed ice

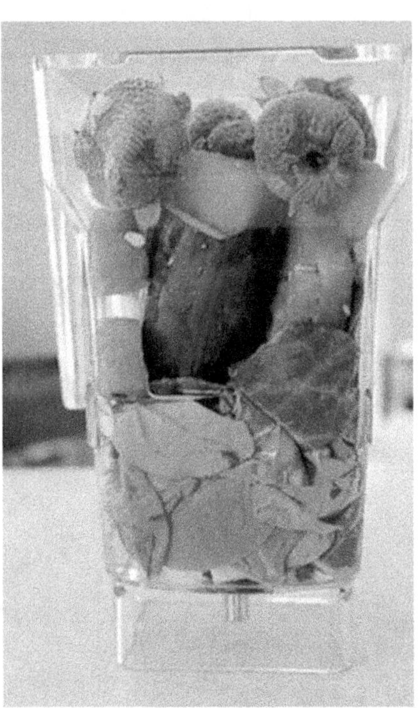

Spinach Blueberries Blackberries Grapefruit Smoothie

- 1 Grapefruit

- 1 cup blackberries

- 1 cup mixed greens (spinach & kale)

- 1/2 cup blueberries

- 1 cup crushed ice

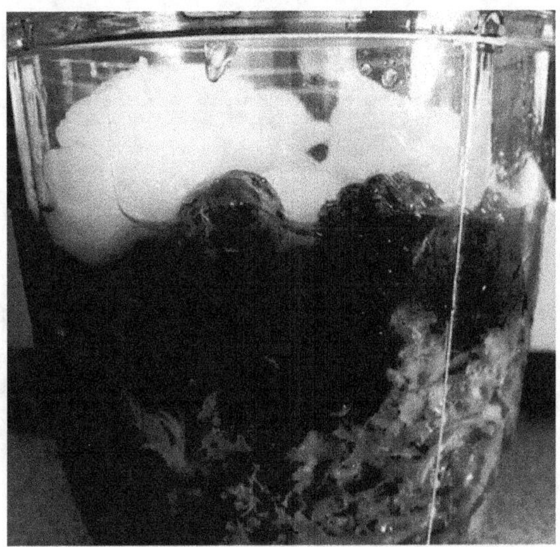

Spinach Almond Milk Banana Apple Smoothie

- 1 cup Almond milk
- 1 banana
- 1 cup spinach
- 1 apple
- 1/2 cup crushed ice

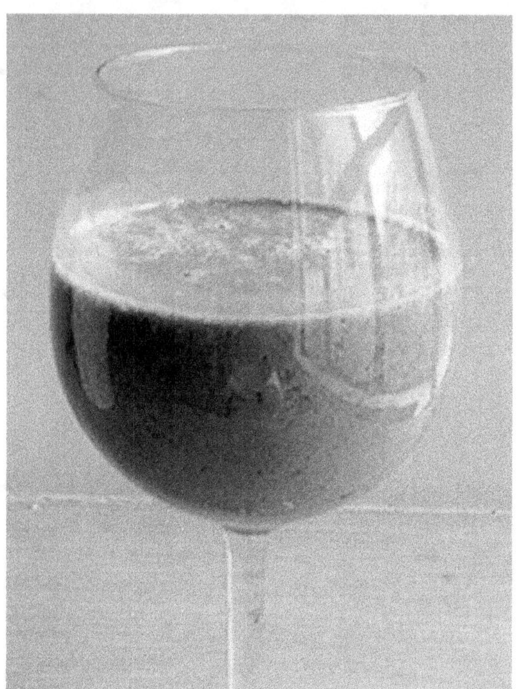

Spinach Apple Banana Avocado Celery Smoothie

* 1 Apple

* 1 banana

* 1 cup Spinach

* 1/2 avocado

* 1 cup Celery

* 1 cup crushed ice

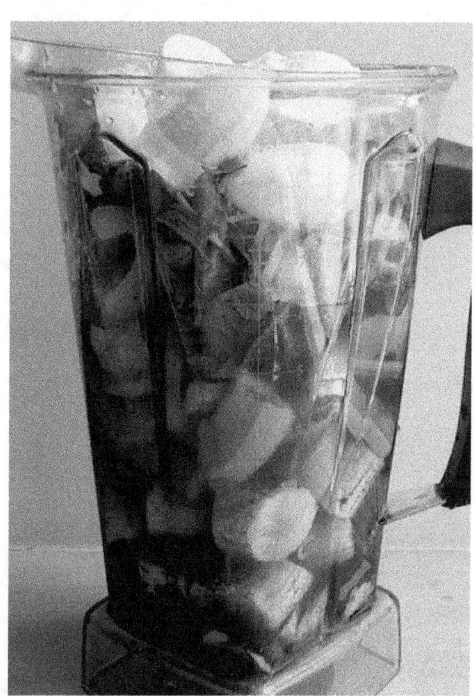

Spinach Banana Strawberries Grapefruit Flax Seeds Smoothie

- 1 cup Strawberries

- 1 banana

- 1 cup Spinach

- 1/2 Grapefruit

- 2 Tbsp. Flax seeds

- 1 cup crushed ice

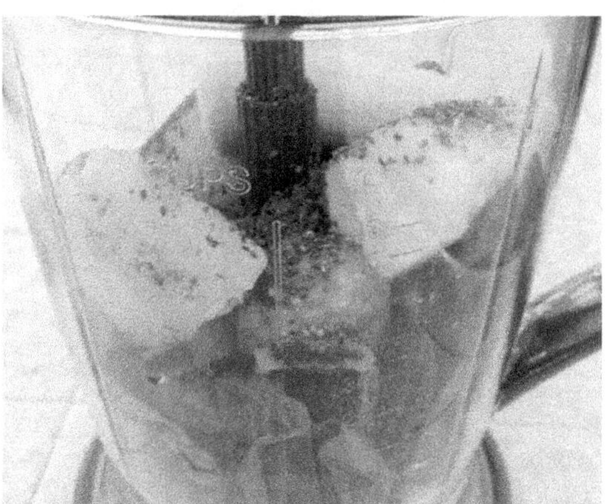

Spinach Blackberry Blueberry Smoothie

- 1 cup frozen blueberries
- 1 cup frozen blackberries
- 1 cup spinach
- 1 cup crushed ice

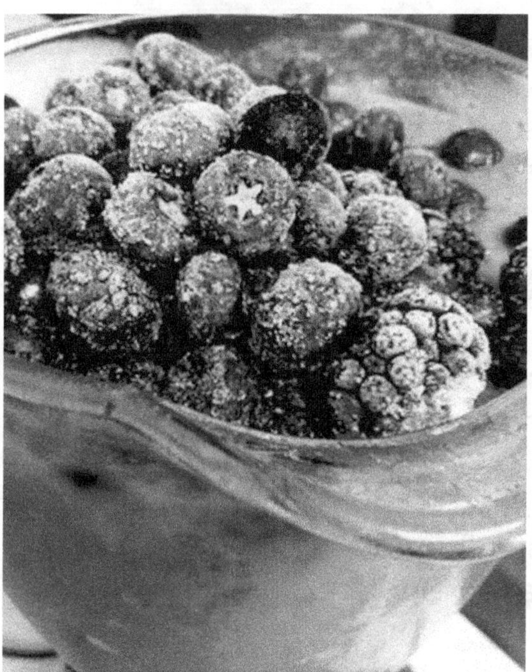

ORAC Value List

ORAC is short for Oxygen Radical Absorbance Capacity. It was developed by the National Institutes of Health in Baltimore.

ORAC units are measurement of the antioxidant capacity of foods. The higher the ORAC value, the more antioxidants the food has.

Foods high in antioxidants lower the risks of cancer and disease.

You'll notice that spices have the most antioxidants. But the ORAC value is measured in dry spices and that is why the values are so high. Common foods such as berries, beans and apples have much fewer antioxidants per gram, because they are full of water. Plus, you can't eat 6 oz. of cloves in one meal, but you can eat 6 oz. of apples. You will notice that e.g. white raisins have higher ORAC value than grape seeds although they are pretty much the same food, but that is because raisins have less water. Every food on this list above value 2 is great. It's better not to pay too much attention to exact ORAC number, just keep eating them all and try to squeeze as much top rated foods as you can. ORAC values in the table are divided per 1000, e.g. Cloves have ORAC rating over 314000, but I slashed 1000 off of each value to keep it easier to compare. Chia seeds are not on this list, but they have value around 6.

#	Item	Value
1	Cloves, ground	314
2	Sumac bran	312
3	Cinnamon, ground	268
4	Sorghum, bran, raw	240
5	Oregano, dried	200
6	Turmeric, ground	159
7	Acai berry, freeze-dried	103
8	Sorghum, bran, black	101
9	Sumac, grain, raw	87
10	Cocoa powder, unsweetened	81
11	Cumin seed	77
12	Maqui berry, powder	75
13	Parsley, dried	74
14	Sorghum, bran, red	71
15	Basil, dried	68
16	Baking chocolate, unsweetened	50
17	Curry powder	49
18	Sorghum, grain, hi-tannin	45
19	Chocolate, dutched powder	40
20	Maqui berry, juice	40

#	Item	Value
21	Sage	32
22	Mustard seed, yellow	29
23	Ginger, ground	29
24	Pepper, black	28
25	Thyme, fresh	27
26	Marjoram, fresh	27
27	Goji berries	25
28	Rice bran, crude	24
29	Chili powder	24
30	Sorghum, grain, black	22
31	Chocolate, dark	21
32	Flax hull lignans	20
33	Chocolate, semisweet	18
34	Pecans	18
35	Paprika	18
36	Chokeberry, raw	16
37	Tarragon, fresh	16
38	Ginger root, raw	15
39	Elderberries, raw	15
40	Sorghum, grain, red	14

41	Peppermint, fresh	14
42	Oregano, fresh	14
43	Walnuts	14
44	Hazelnuts	10
45	Cranberries, raw	10
46	Pears, dried	9
47	Savory, fresh	9
48	Artichokes	9
49	Kidney beans, red	8
50	Pink beans	8
51	Black beans	8
52	Pistachio nuts	8
53	Currants	8
54	Pinto beans	8
55	Plums	8
56	Chocolate, milk chocolate	8
57	Lentils	7
58	Agave, dried	7
59	Apples, dried	7
60	Garlic powder	7

61	Blueberries	7
62	Prunes	7
63	Sorghum, bran, white	6
64	Lemon balm, leaves	6
65	Soybeans	6
66	Onion powder	6
67	Blackberries	5
68	Garlic, raw	5
69	Cilantro leaves	5
70	Wine, Cabernet Sauvignon	5
71	Raspberries	5
72	Basil, fresh	5
73	Almonds	4
74	Dill weed	4
75	Cowpeas	4
76	Apples, red delicious	4
77	Peaches, dried	4
78	Raisins, white	4
79	Apples, granny smith	4
80	Dates	4

81	Wine, red	4
82	Strawberries	4
83	Peanut butter, smooth	3
84	Currants, red	3
85	Figs	3
86	Cherries	3
87	Gooseberries	3
88	Apricots, dried	3
89	Peanuts, all types	3
90	Cabbage, red	3
91	Broccoli	3
92	Apples	3
93	Raisins	3
94	Pears	3
95	Agave	3
96	Blueberry juice	3
97	Cardamom	2,7
98	Guava	2,5
99	Lettuce, red leaf	2,38
100	Concord grape juice	2,37

101	Cereals, ready-to-eat, corn flakes	2,36
102	Juice, Pomegranate, 100%	2,34
103	Cereals, oats, instant, fortified, plain, dry	2,31
104	Cereals ready-to-eat, granola, low-fat, with raisins	2,29
105	Cabbage, red, raw	2,25
106	Apples, Golden Delicious, raw, without skin	2,21
107	Sorghum, grain, white	2,20
108	Radish seeds, sprouted, raw	2,18
109	Cereals ready-to-eat, oat bran	2,18
110	Cereals ready-to-eat, toasted oatmeal	2,18
111	Cereals, oats, quick, uncooked	2,17
112	Asparagus, raw	2,15
113	Cereals ready-to-eat, oatmeal, toasted squares	2,14
114	Sweet potato, cooked, baked in skin, without salt	2,12
115	Bread, butternut whole grain	2,10
116	Chives, raw	2,09
117	Cabbage, savoy, cooked, boiled, drained, without salt	2,05
118	Prune juice, canned	2,04
119	Guava, red-fleshed	1,99
120	Applesauce, canned, unsweetened, without added ascorbic acid	1,97

121	Bread, pumpernickel	1,96
122	Nuts, cashew nuts, raw	1,95
123	Beet greens, raw	1,95
124	Avocados, Hass, raw	1,93
125	Pears, green cultivars, with peel, raw	1,91
126	Rocket, raw	1,90
127	Oranges, raw, navels	1,82
128	Peaches, raw	1,81
129	Juice, red grape	1,79
130	Cabbage, black, cooked	1,77
131	Beets, raw	1,77
132	Pears, red anjou, raw	1,75
133	Snacks, popcorn, air-popped	1,74
134	Radishes, raw	1,74
135	Cereals, oats, old fashioned, uncooked	1,71
136	Tortilla chips, reduced fat, Olestra - TEMPORARY	1,70
137	Nuts, macadamia nuts, dry roasted, without salt added	1,70
138	Spinach, frozen, chopped or leaf, unprepared	1,69
139	Potatoes, Russet, flesh and skin, baked	1,68
140	Asparagus, cooked, boiled, drained	1,64

141	Tangerines, (mandarin oranges), raw	1,62
142	Broccoli raab, cooked	1,55
143	Grapefruit, raw, pink and red, all areas	1,55
144	Onions, red, raw	1,52
145	Beans, navy, mature seeds, raw	1,52
146	Cereals ready-to-eat, QUAKER, QUAKER OAT LIFE, plain	1,52
147	Spinach, raw	1,52
148	Alfalfa seeds, sprouted, raw	1,51
149	Juice, Cranberry/Concord grape	1,48
150	Lettuce, green leaf, raw	1,45
151	Lettuce, butterhead (includes boston and bibb types), raw	1,42
152	Bread, mixed-grain (includes whole-grain, 7-grain)	1,42
153	Nuts, brazilnuts, dried, unblanched	1,42
154	Broccoli, raw	1,36
155	Potatoes, red, flesh and skin, baked	1,33
156	Potatoes, russet, flesh and skin, raw	1,32
157	Bread, Oatnut	1,32
158	Cereals ready-to-eat, wheat, shredded, plain, sugar and salt free	1,30
159	Parsley, raw	1,30
160	Milk, chocolate, fluid, commercial, reduced fat	1,26

161	Grapes, red, raw	1,26
162	Tea, green, brewed	1,25
163	Agave, raw (Southwest)	1,25
164	Grapefruit juice, white, raw	1,24
165	Lemon juice, raw	1,23
166	Onions, yellow, sauteed	1,22
167	Kiwi, gold, raw	1,21
168	Olive oil, extra-virgin	1,15
169	Potatoes, white, flesh and skin, baked	1,14
170	Tea, brewed, prepared with tap water	1,13
171	Grapes, white or green, raw	1,12
172	Apricots, raw	1,12
173	Potatoes, red, flesh and skin, raw	1,10
174	Potatoes, white, flesh and skin, raw	1,06
175	Onions, raw	1,03
176	Alcoholic beverage, wine, table, rose	1,01
177	Mangos, raw	1,00
178	Juice, strawberry	1,00
179	Sauce, ready-to-serve, salsa	1,00
180	Peppers, sweet, orange, raw	0,98

181	Peppers, sweet, yellow, raw	0,97
182	Lettuce, cos or romaine, raw	0,96
183	Soybeans, mature seeds, sprouted, raw	0,96
184	Eggplant, raw	0,93
185	Peppers, sweet, green, raw	0,92
186	Beans, pinto, mature seeds, cooked, boiled, without salt	0,90
187	Sweet potato, raw, unprepared	0,90
188	Pineapple, raw, extra sweet variety	0,88
189	Kiwi fruit, (chinese gooseberries), fresh, raw	0,88
190	Bananas, raw	0,88
191	Juice, cranberrry, 100% - cranberry blend, red	0,87
192	Onions, white, raw	0,86
193	Cabbage, cooked, boiled, drained, without salt	0,86
194	Chickpeas (garbanzo beans, bengal gram), mature seeds, raw	0,85
195	Peppers, sweet, red, sauteed	0,85
196	Raisins, white, fresh (purchased in Italy)	0,83
197	Cauliflower, raw	0,83
198	Lime juice, raw	0,82
199	Grape juice, white	0,79
200	Peppers, sweet, red, raw	0,79

201	Olive oil, extra-virgin, w/parsley, home prepared	0,77
202	Sweet potato, cooked, boiled, without skin	0,77
203	Beans, snap, green, raw	0,76
204	Nectarines, raw	0,75
205	Peas, yellow, mature seeds, raw	0,74
206	Chilchen (Red Berry Beverage) (Navajo)	0,74
207	Corn, sweet, yellow, raw	0,73
208	Orange juice, raw	0,73
209	Pear juice, all varieties	0,70
210	Peppers, sweet, yellow, grilled	0,69
211	Tomato products, canned, sauce	0,69
212	Mush, blue corn with ash (Navajo)	0,68
213	Olive oil, extra-virgin, w/basil, home prepared	0,68
214	Carrots, raw	0,67
215	Cauliflower, cooked, boiled, drained, without salt	0,62
216	Nuts, pine nuts, dried	0,62
217	Peppers, sweet, green, sauteed	0,62
218	Onions, sweet, raw	0,61
219	Peas, green, frozen, unprepared	0,60
220	Catsup	0,58
221	Pineapple juice, canned, unsweetened, without added ascorbic acid	0,57
222	Vinegar, Apple	0,56
223	Pineapple, raw, traditional varieties	0,56
224	Olive oil, extra-virgin, w/garlic, home prepared	0,56
225	Vegetable juice cocktail, canned	0,55
226	Tomatoes, plum, raw	0,55
227	Peas, split, mature seeds, raw	0,52
228	Corn, sweet, yellow, frozen, kernels cut off cob, unprepared	0,52
229	Cabbage, raw	0,51
230	Celery, raw	0,50
231	Broccoli, frozen, spears, unprepared	0,50
232	Leeks, (bulb and lower leaf-portion), raw	0,49
233	Tomato juice, canned, with salt added	0,49
234	Cocoa mix, powder	0,49
235	Pumpkin, raw	0,48
236	Spices, poppy seed	0,48
237	Lettuce, iceberg (includes crisphead types), raw	0,44
238	Carrots, baby, raw	0,44
239	Peaches, canned, heavy syrup, drained	0,44
240	Babyfood, juice, pear	0,41
241	Corn, sweet, yellow, canned, brine pack, regular pack, solids and liquids	0,41

242	Vinegar, Red wine	0,41
243	Apple juice, canned or bottled, unsweetened, without added ascorbic acid	0,41
244	Tomatoes, red, ripe, cooked	0,41
245	Squash, winter, butternut, raw	0,40
246	Alcoholic beverage, wine, table, white	0,39
247	Pineapple, raw, all varieties	0,39
248	Tomatoes, red, ripe, raw, year round average	0,37
249	Carrots, cooked, boiled, drained, without salt	0,32
250	Melons, cantaloupe, raw	0,32
251	Fennel, bulb, raw	0,31
252	Beans, snap, green variety, canned, regular pack, solids and liquids	0,29
253	Vinegar, Apple and Honey	0,27
254	Eggplant, cooked, boiled, drained, without salt	0,25
255	Beans, lima, immature seeds, canned, regular pack, solids and liquids	0,24
256	Melons, honeydew, raw	0,24
257	Juice, cranberry, white	0,23
258	Vinegar, Honey	0,23
259	Olive oil, extra-virgin, w/garlic and red hot peppers, home prepared	0,22
260	Cucumber, with peel, raw	0,21

261	Squash, summer, zucchini, includes skin, raw	0,18
262	Watermelon, raw	0,14
263	Cucumber, peeled, raw	0,13
264	Oil, peanut, salad or cooking	0,11
265	Limes, raw	0,08